The
Mighty
Bug

Written By
Mary D Wynn

Illustrated By
Len Peralta

Published By
Wynnstreet Press
Redford, Michigan
ISBN: 978-1-7375242-0-5

First Edition, 2021

TO MY MOM AND DAD:
Two of the most gifted storytellers in the world.

AND TO MY DAUGHTERS:
Follow your heart and dreams, and along the way,
choose to do the right thing.

A powerful sneeze tore through the air!
It blew them all out of their chair.
Mighty Bug looked around in despair.
Where was his family?
They were nowhere.

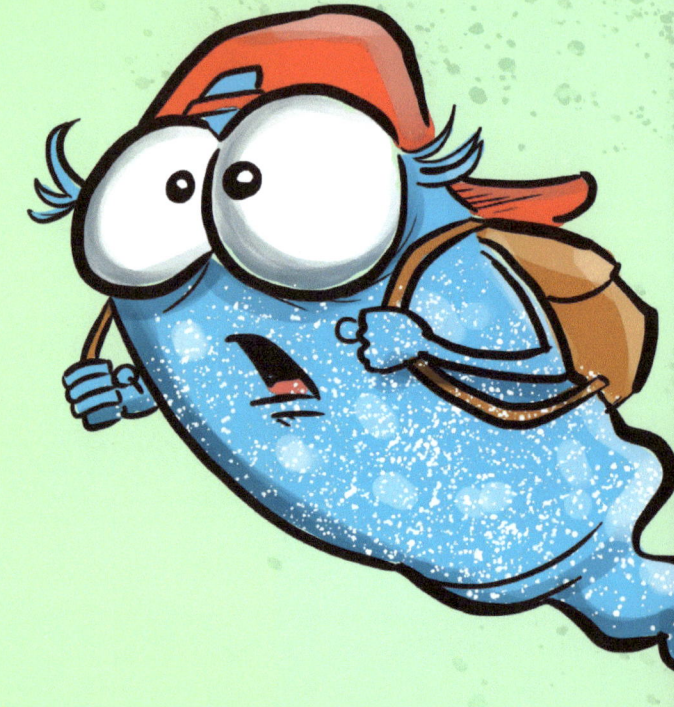

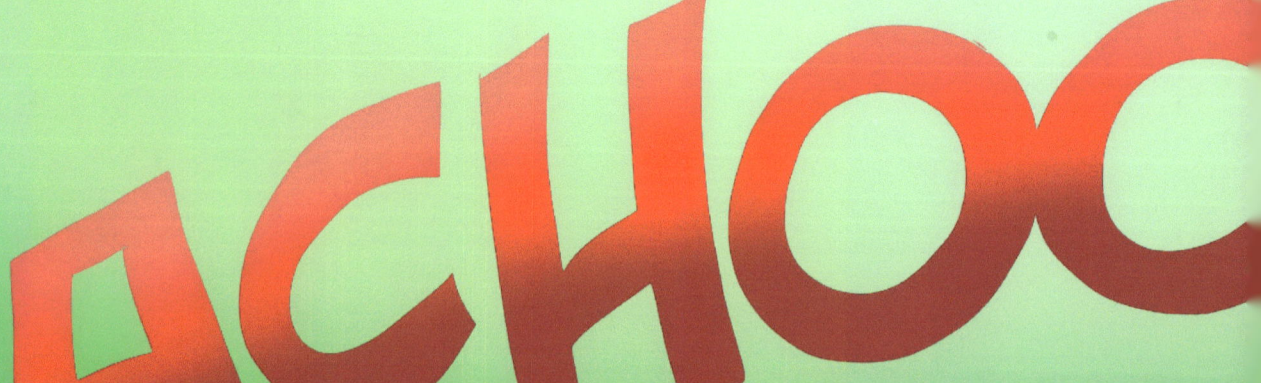

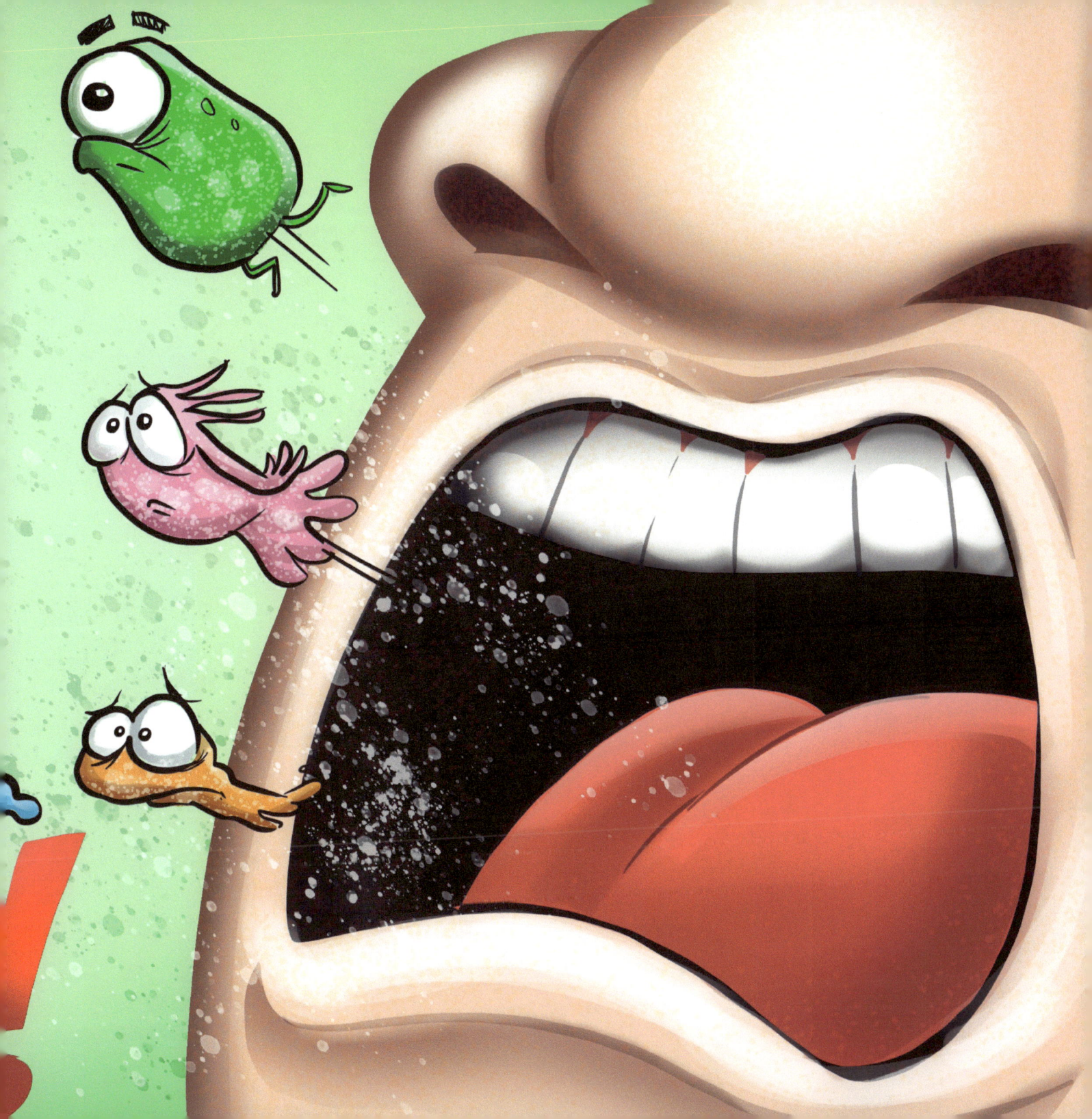

Mighty Bug felt sad and alone.

Without his family.

Away from his home.

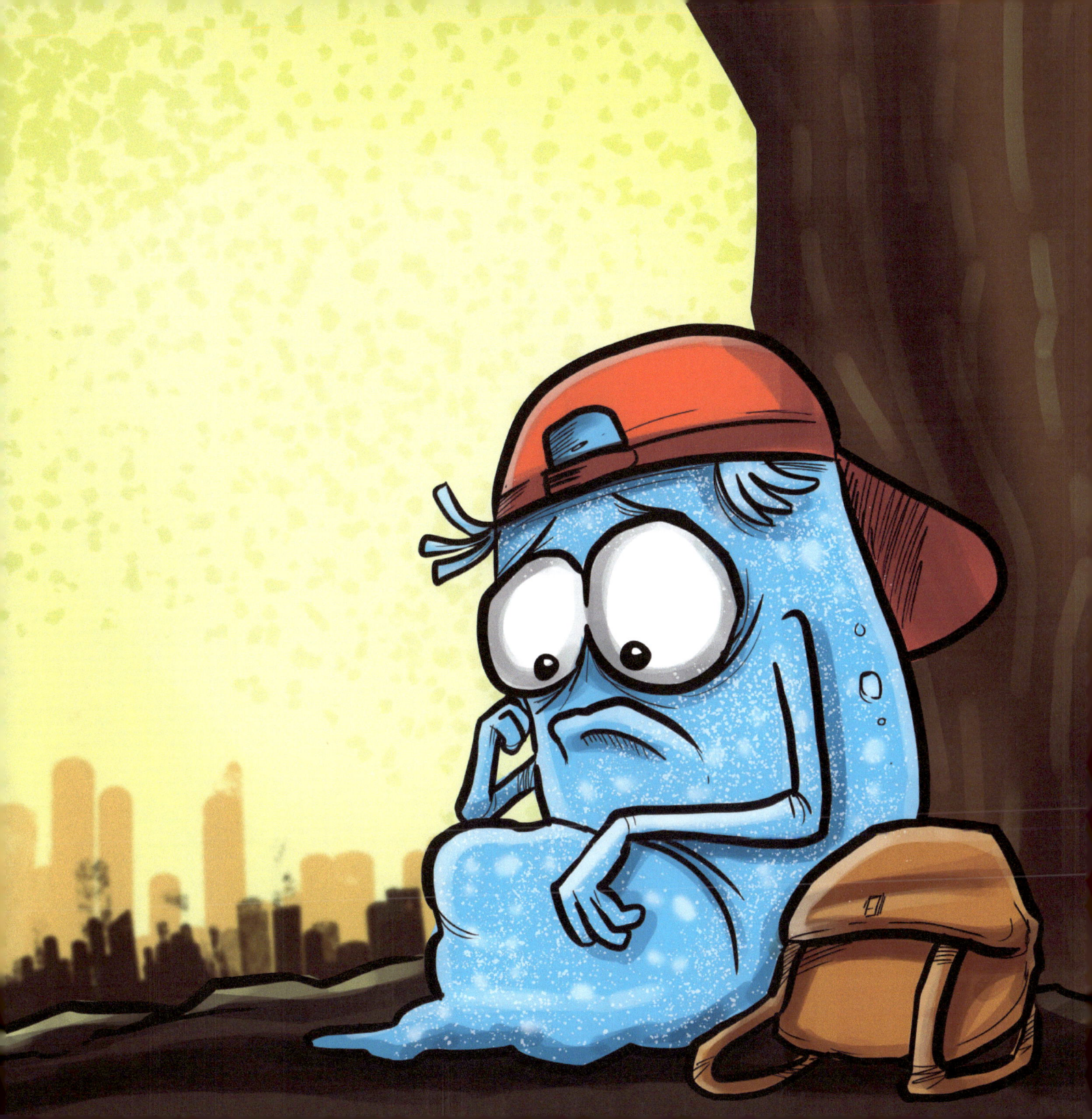

Mighty Bug studied a map and thought of a plan.
He'd find a way to see his family again.

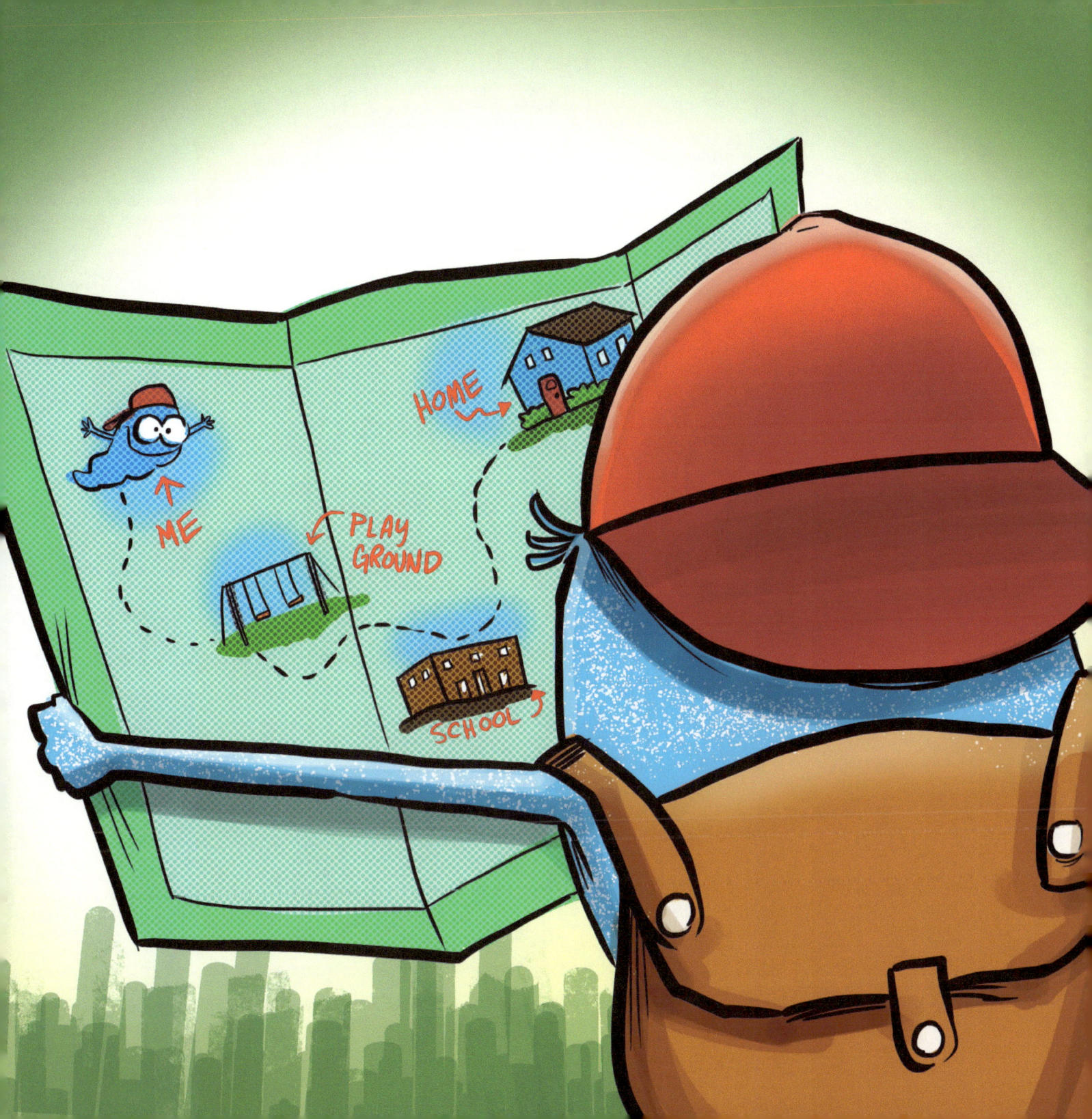

He was determined to be his best.
So he went to bed early and got plenty of rest.
When morning came, he looked for a hand.
He waited patiently for his chance to land.

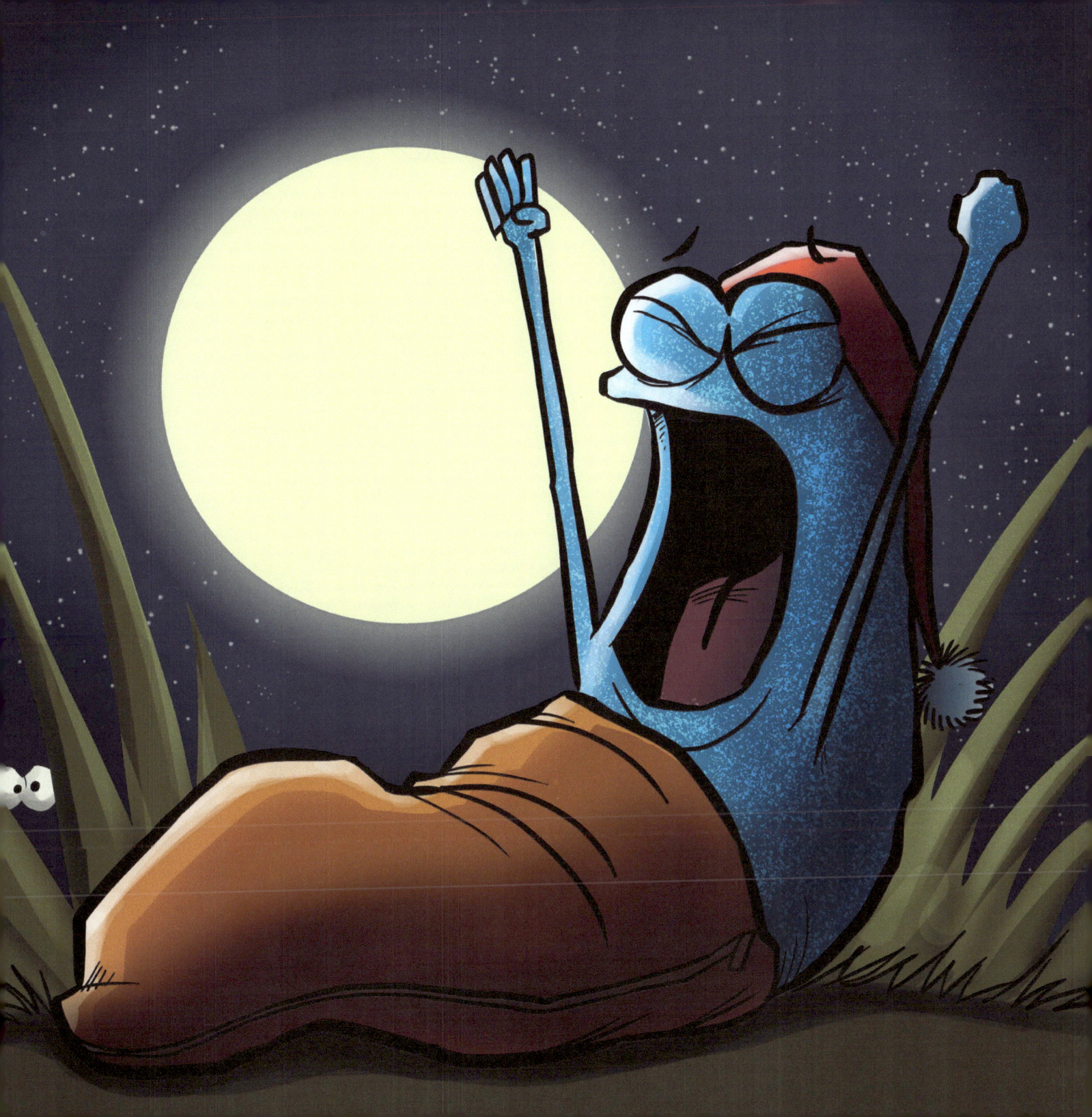

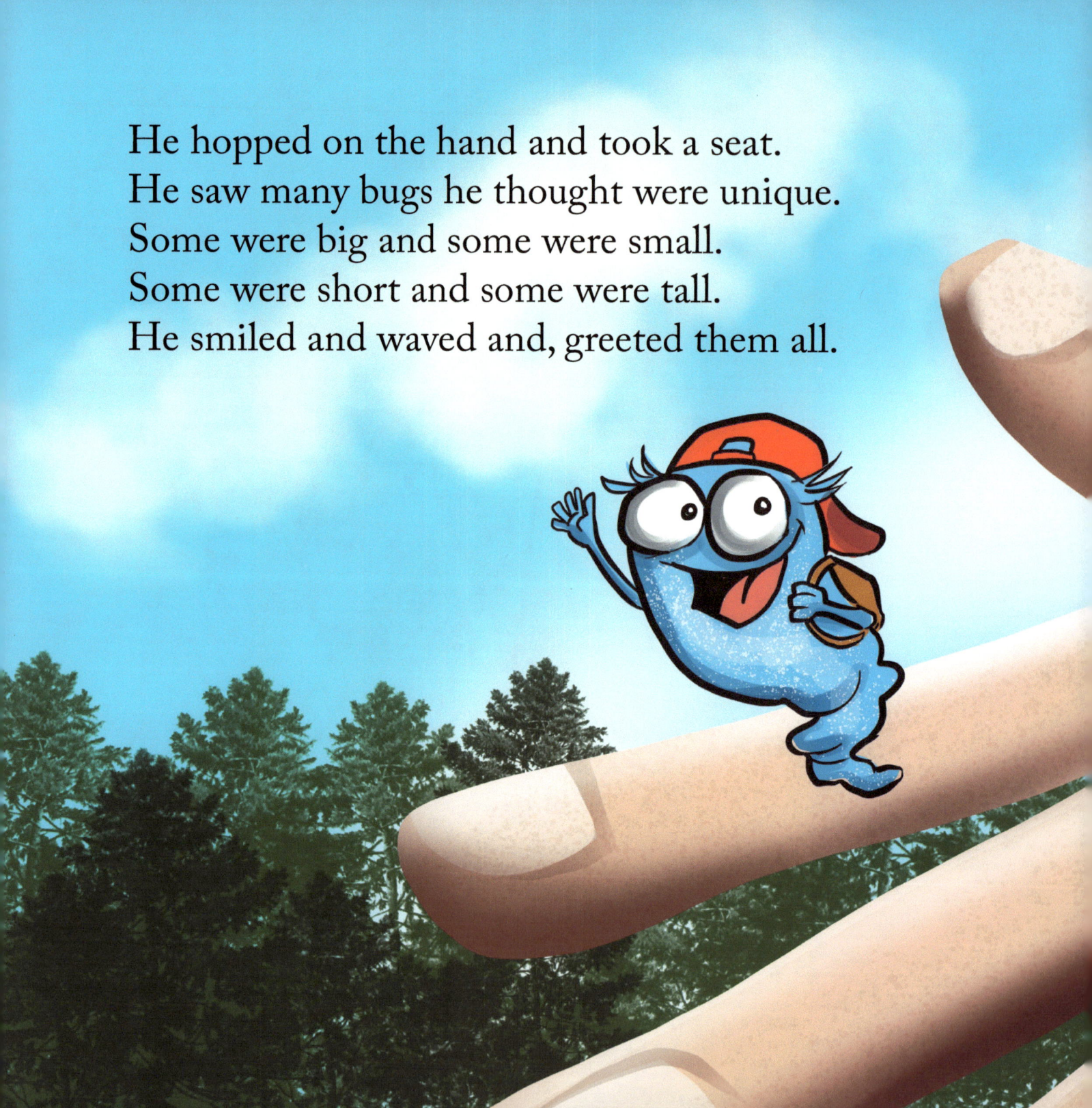

He hopped on the hand and took a seat.
He saw many bugs he thought were unique.
Some were big and some were small.
Some were short and some were tall.
He smiled and waved and, greeted them all.

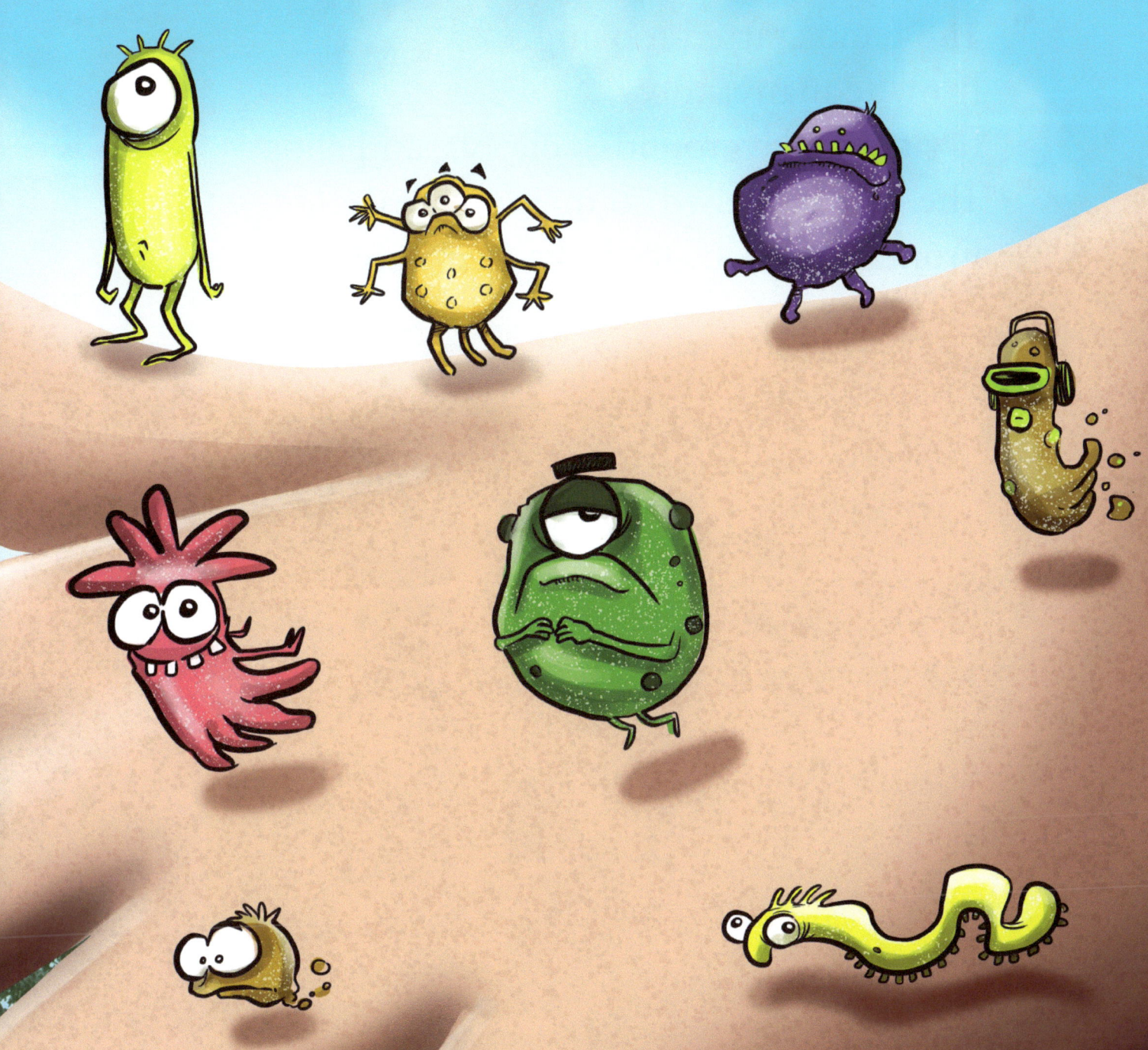

The hand started moving.
It made many stops.
It visited playgrounds, schools, and shops.
The hand touched so many places!
From doorknobs to desks then tables and faces.

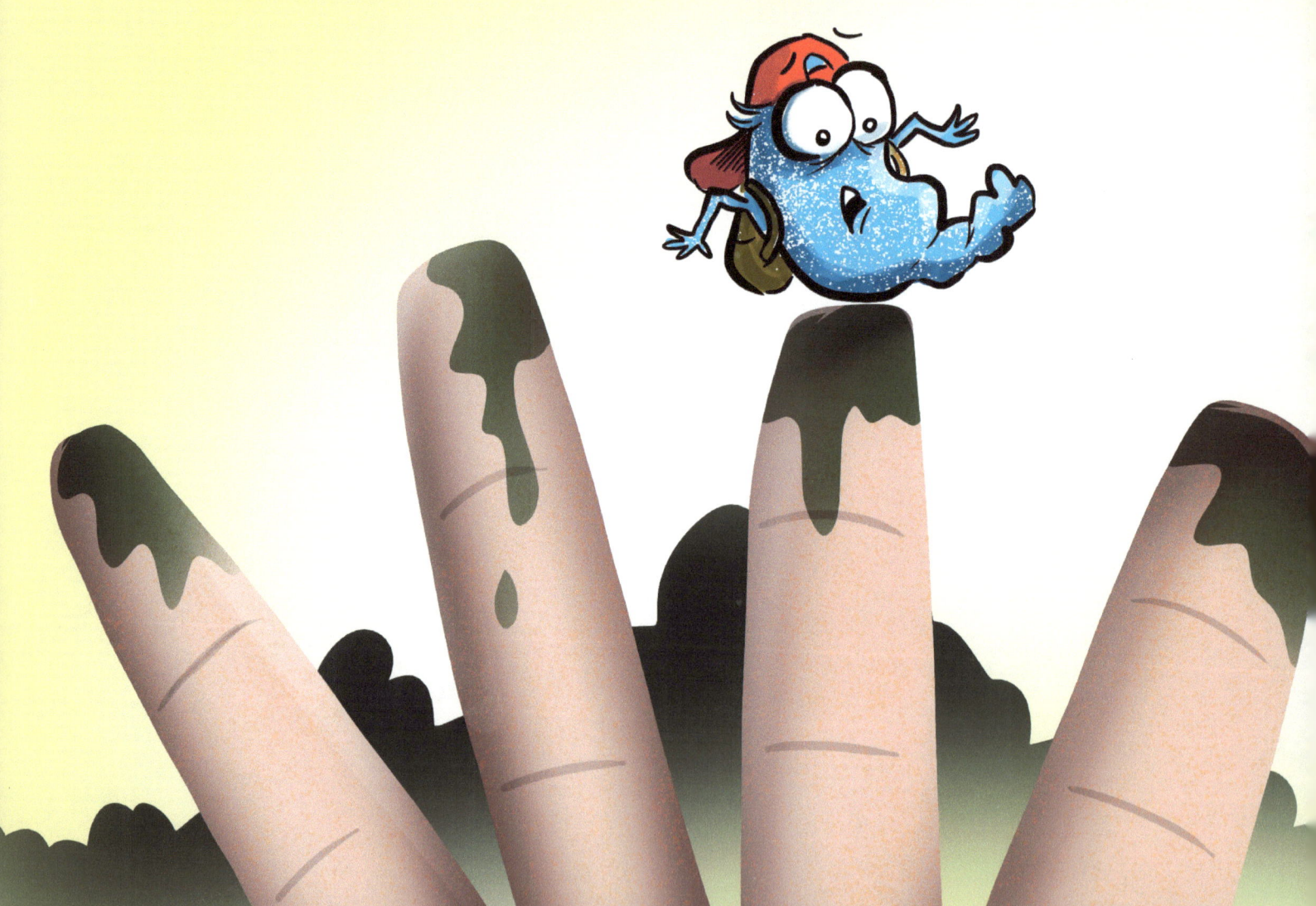

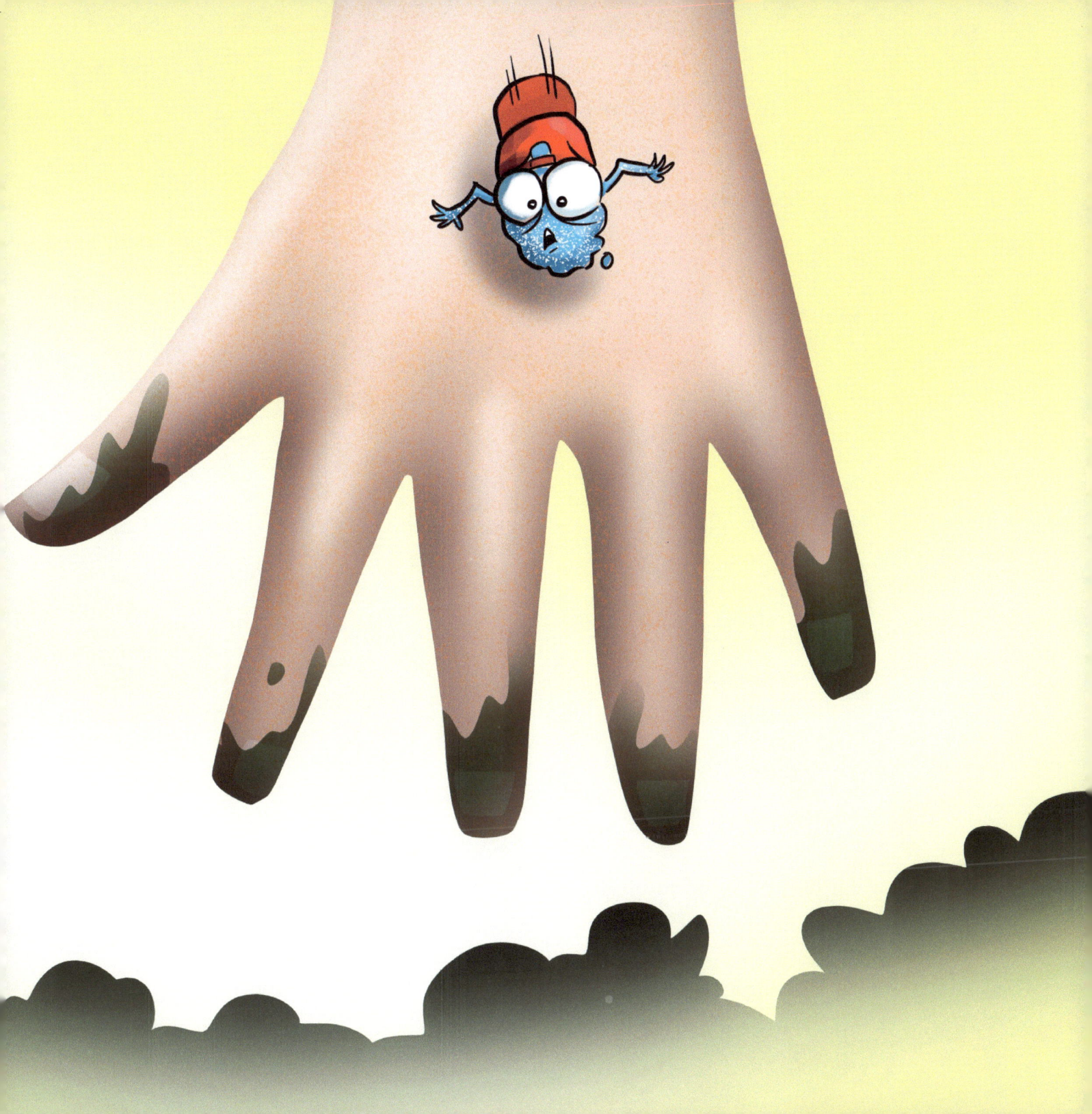

Some bugs hopped on while others jumped off.
They hopped on with a sneeze.
They jumped off with a cough.
Mighty Bug held tight and stayed strong.
He didn't jump with the others; he just stayed on.

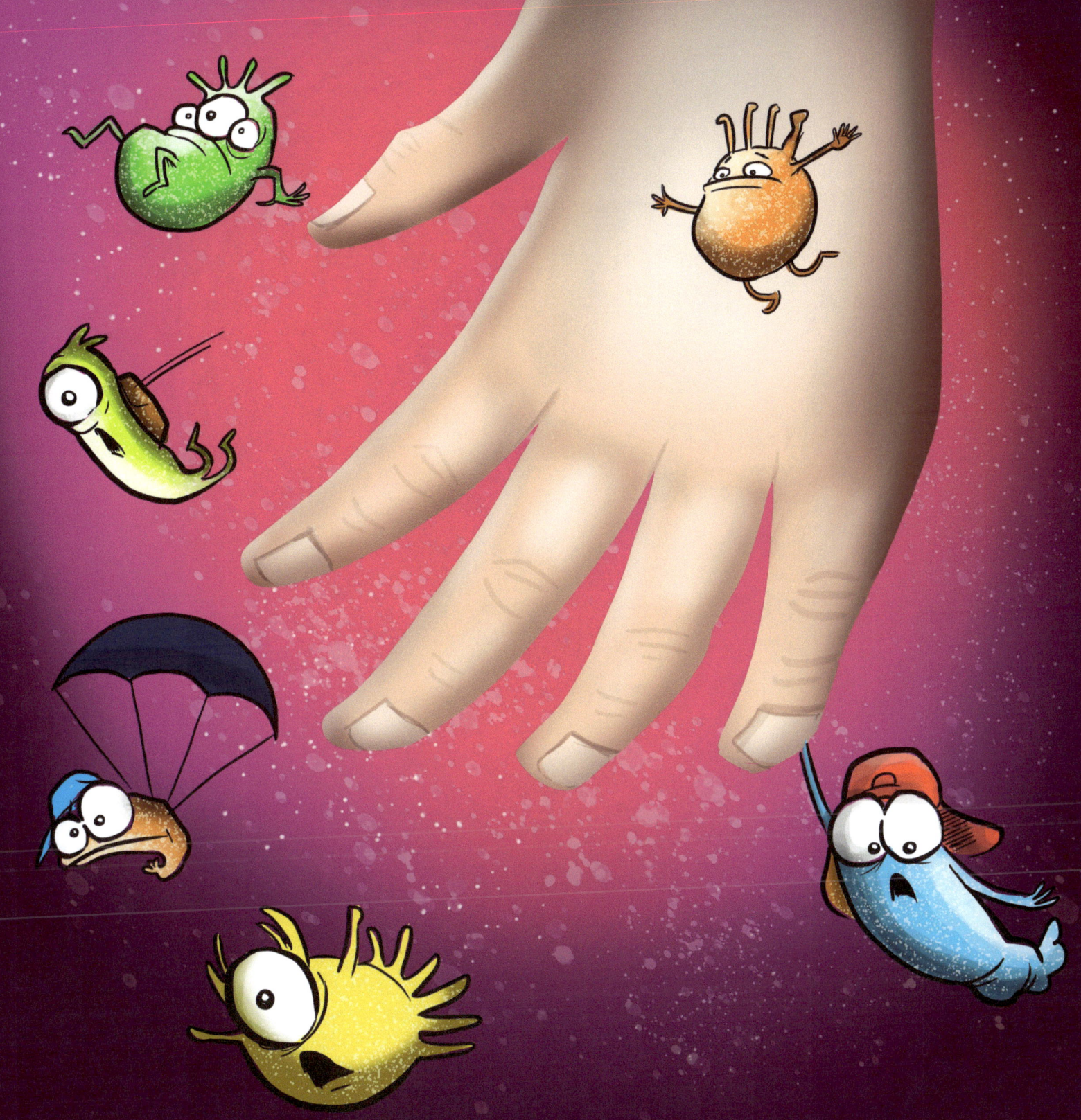

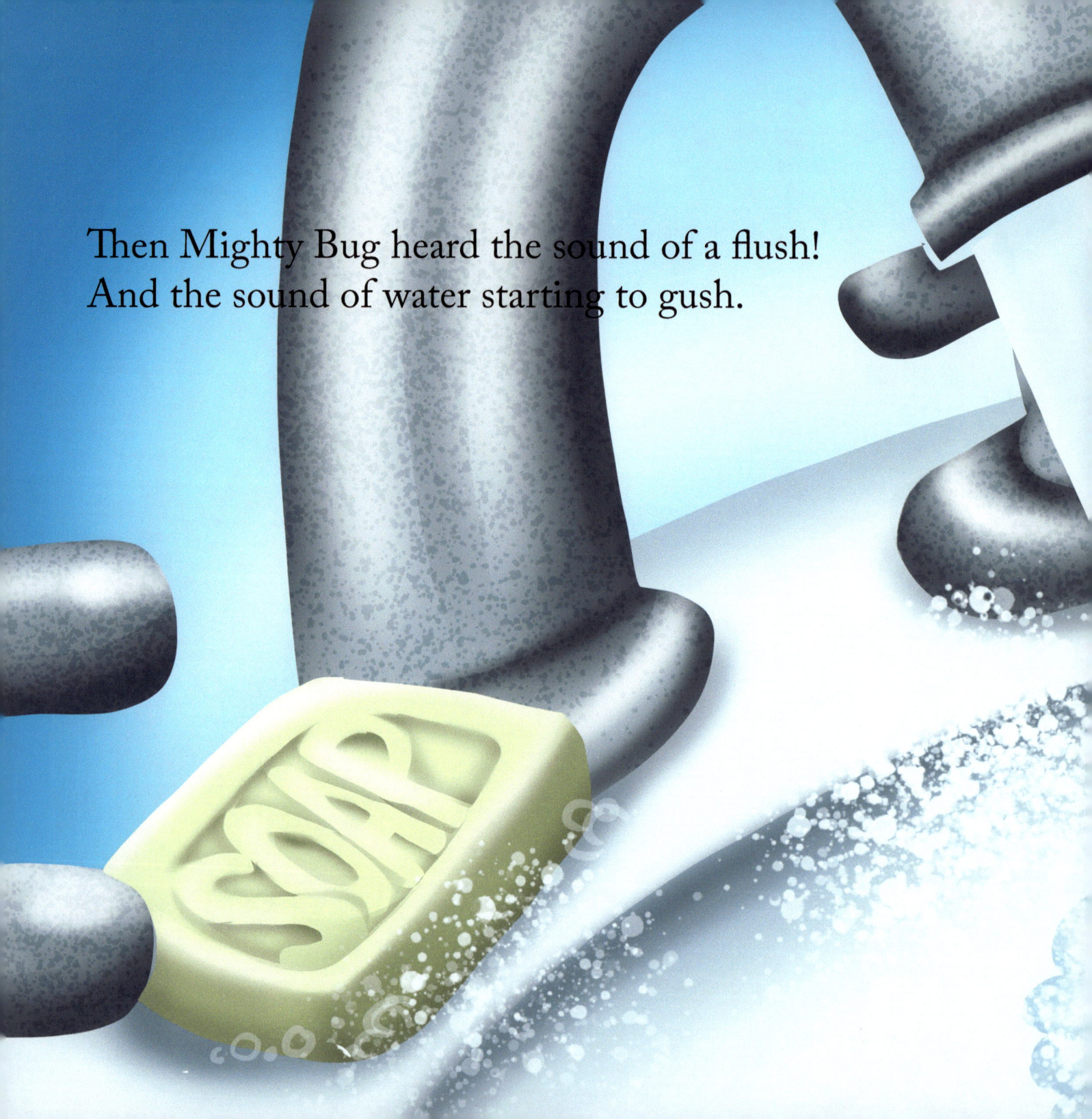

Then Mighty Bug heard the sound of a flush!
And the sound of water starting to gush.

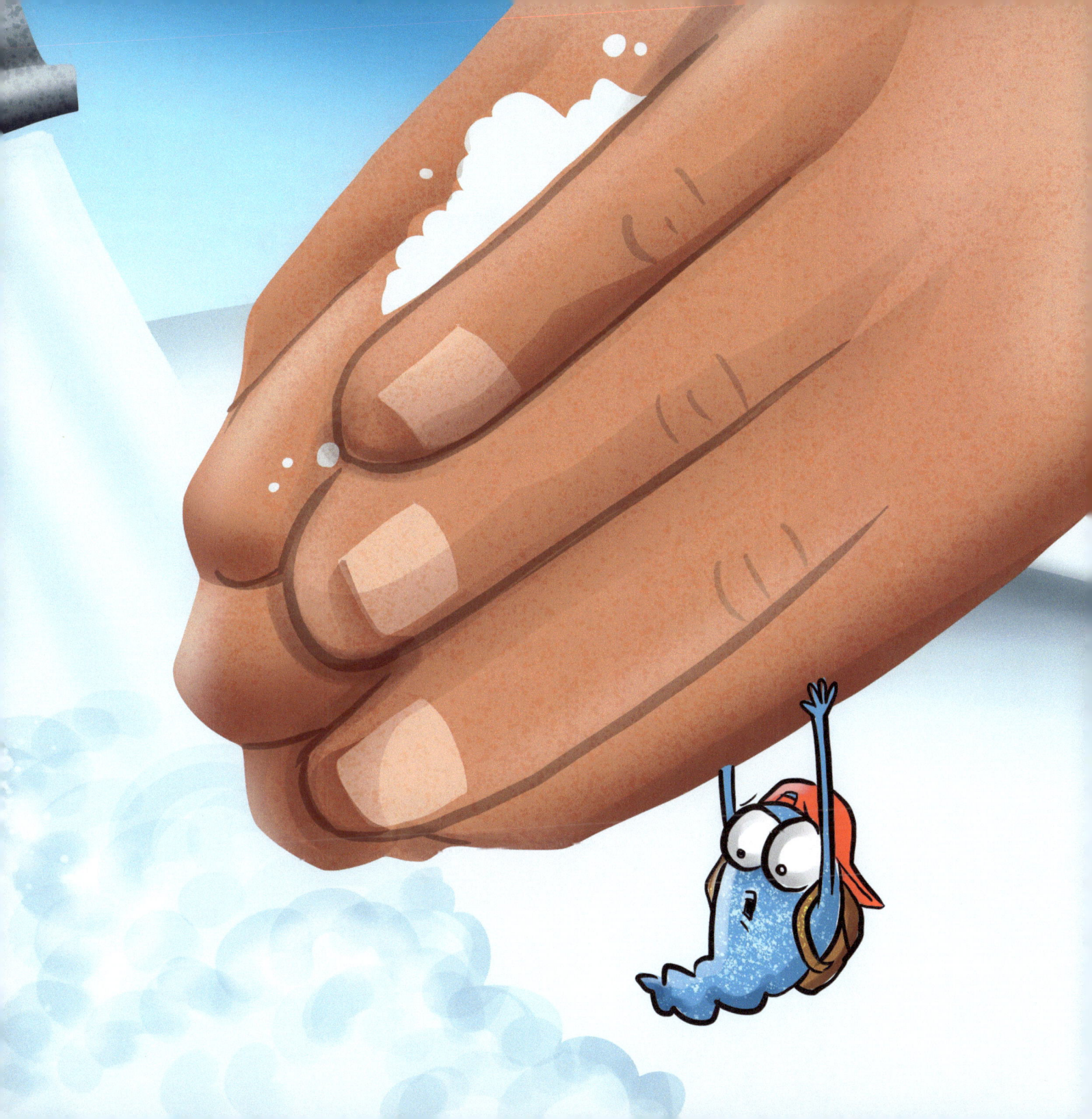

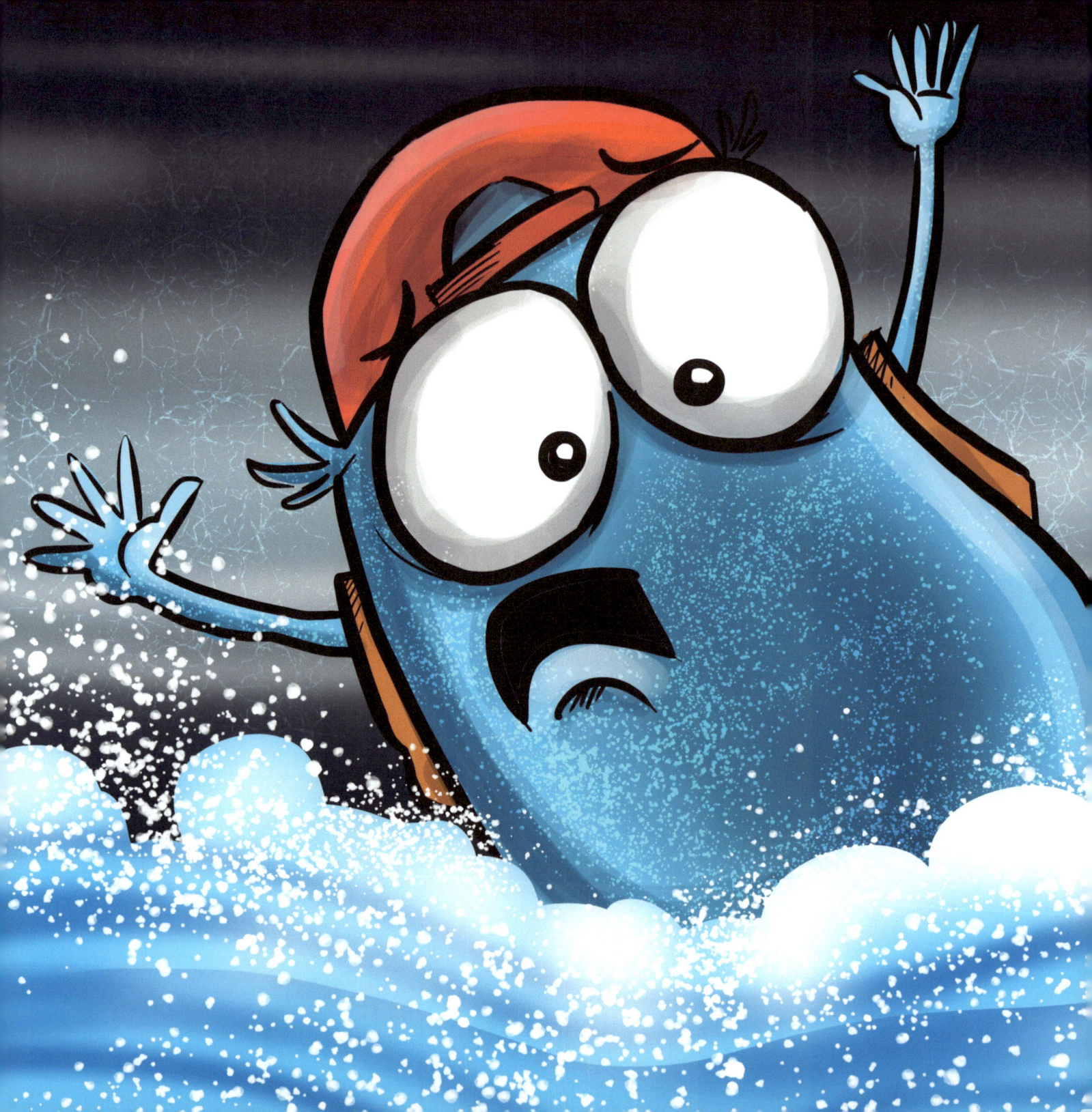

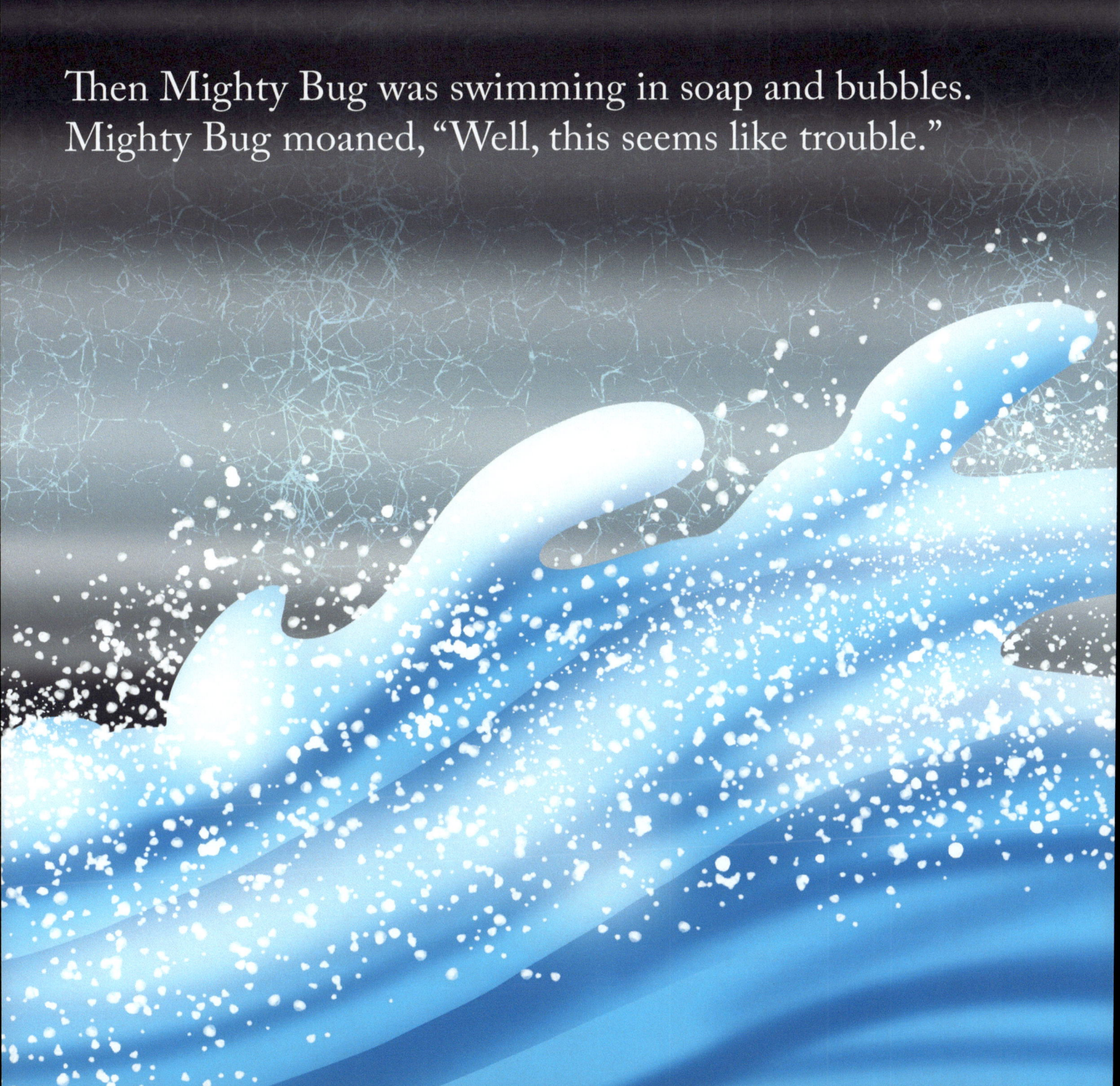

Then Mighty Bug was swimming in soap and bubbles. Mighty Bug moaned, "Well, this seems like trouble."

His vision blurred.
He could not see!
His body felt hot and quite shaky.

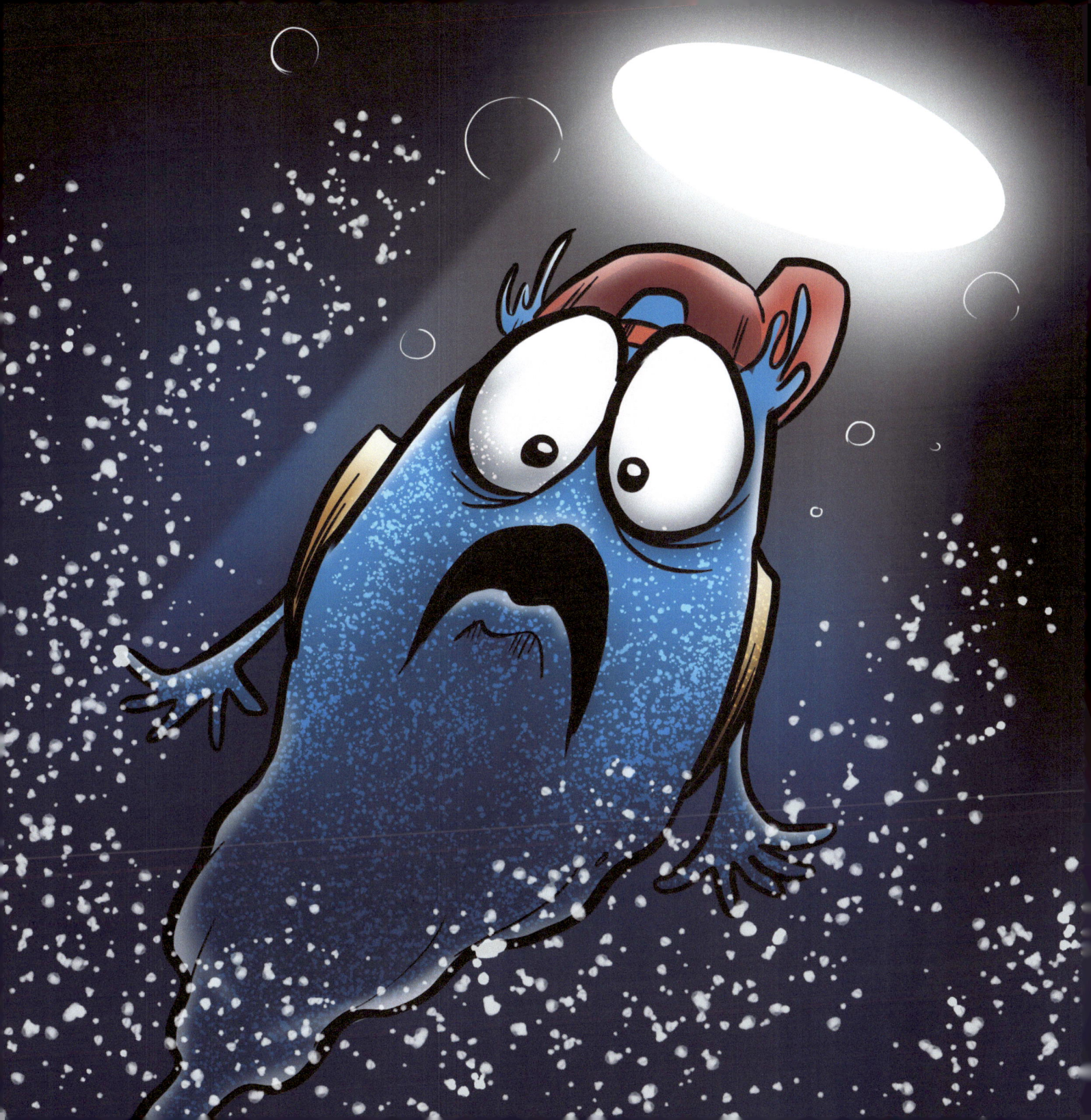

Mighty Bug got dizzy and fell from the hand.
This journey was not turning out like he'd planned.
He swirled around and down into funnel.
Then, he slid into a long scary tunnel.

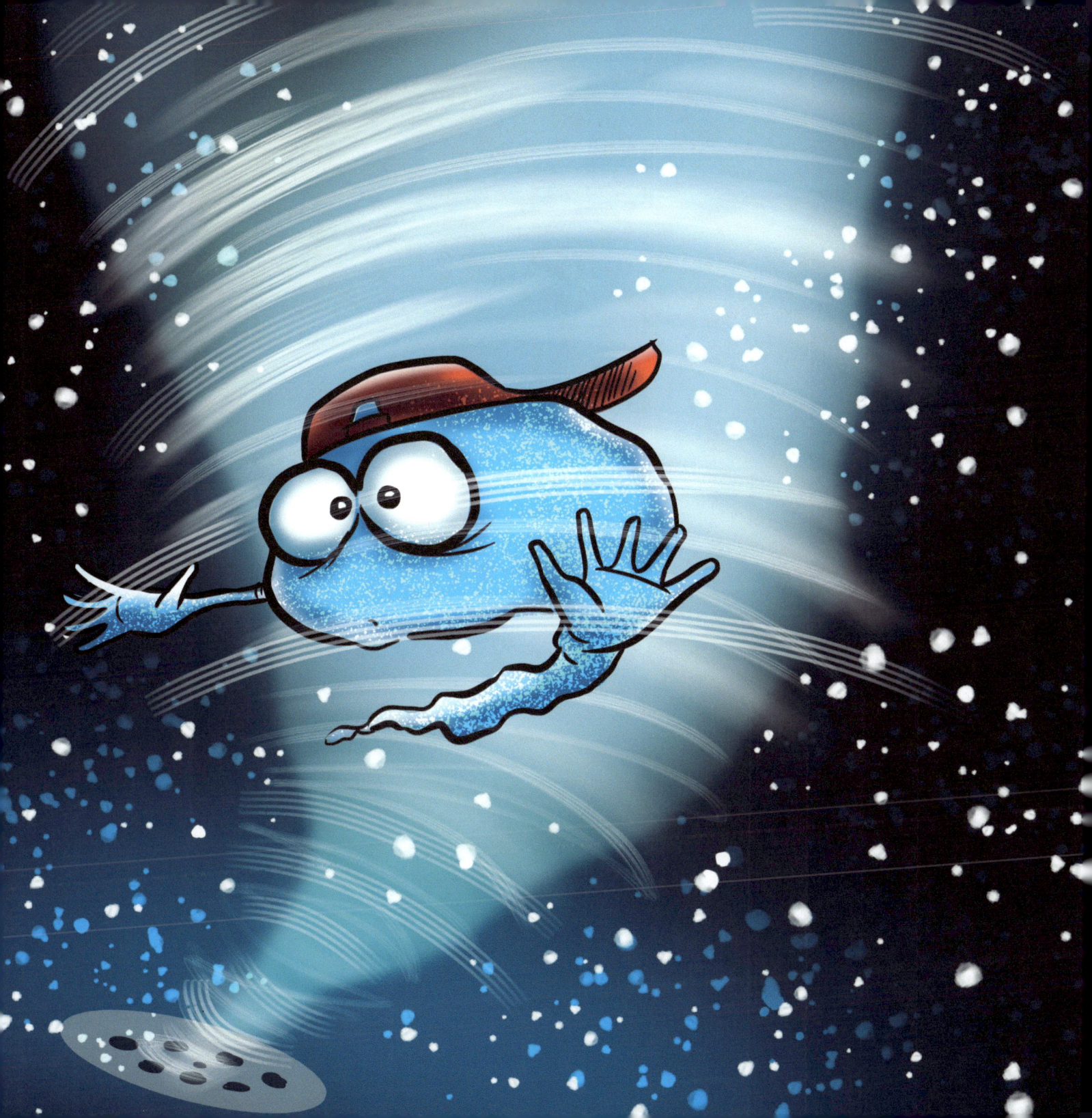

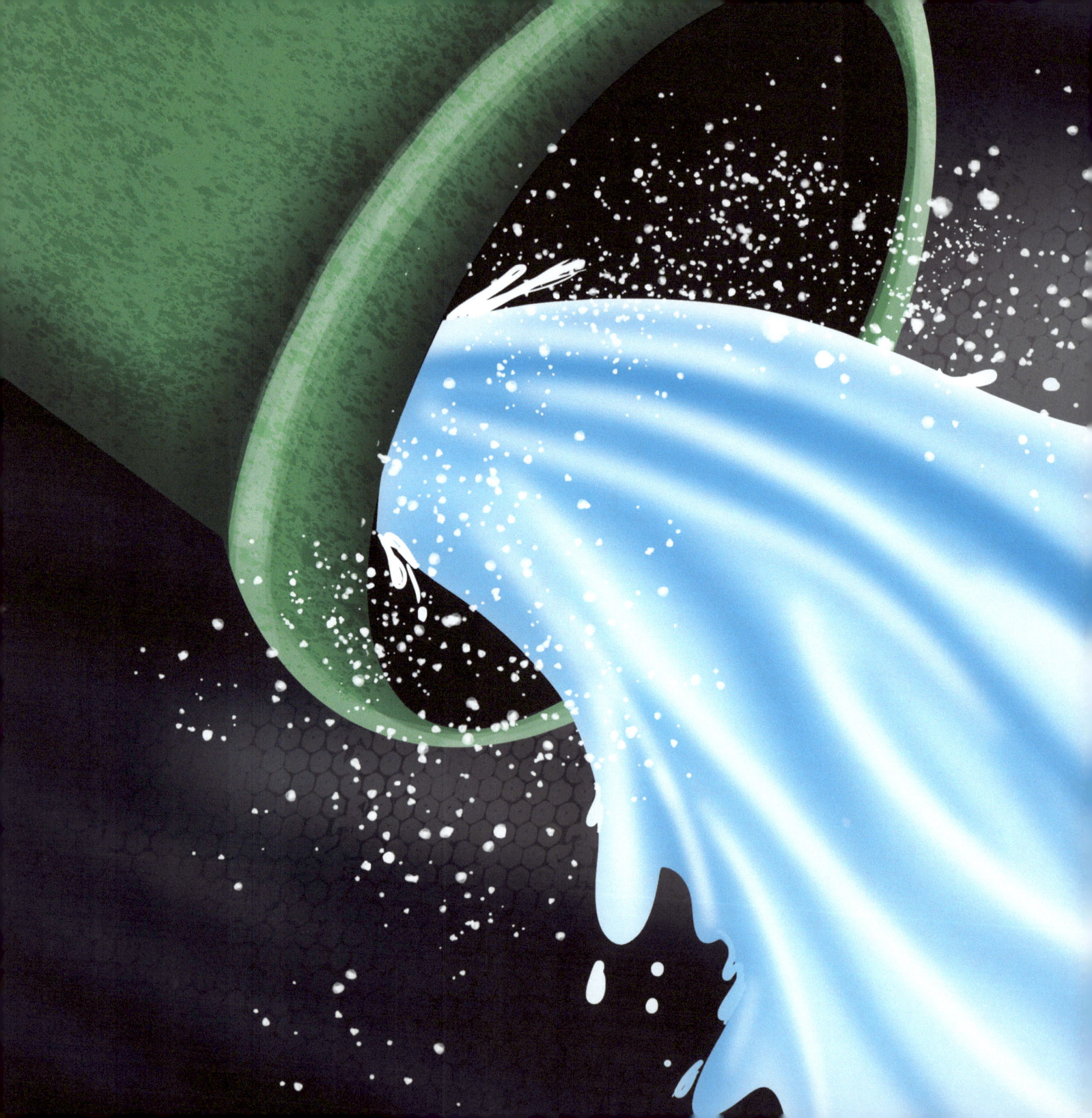

Whoosh! He blasted out, all cold and wet!
Mighty Bug felt scared and started to fret.

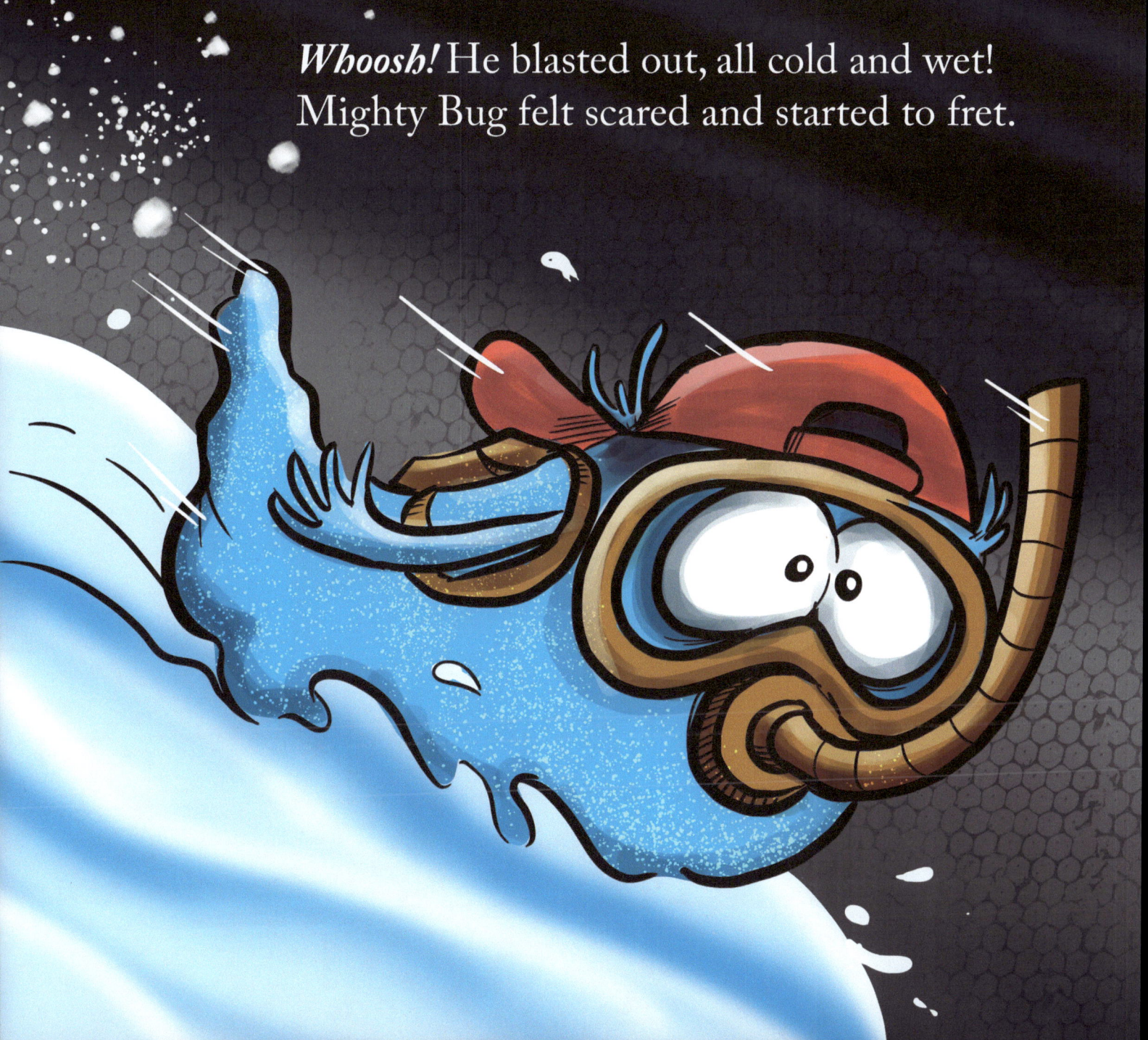

Then he heard the sounds of laughter and cheer.
He looked up and realized his family was near.

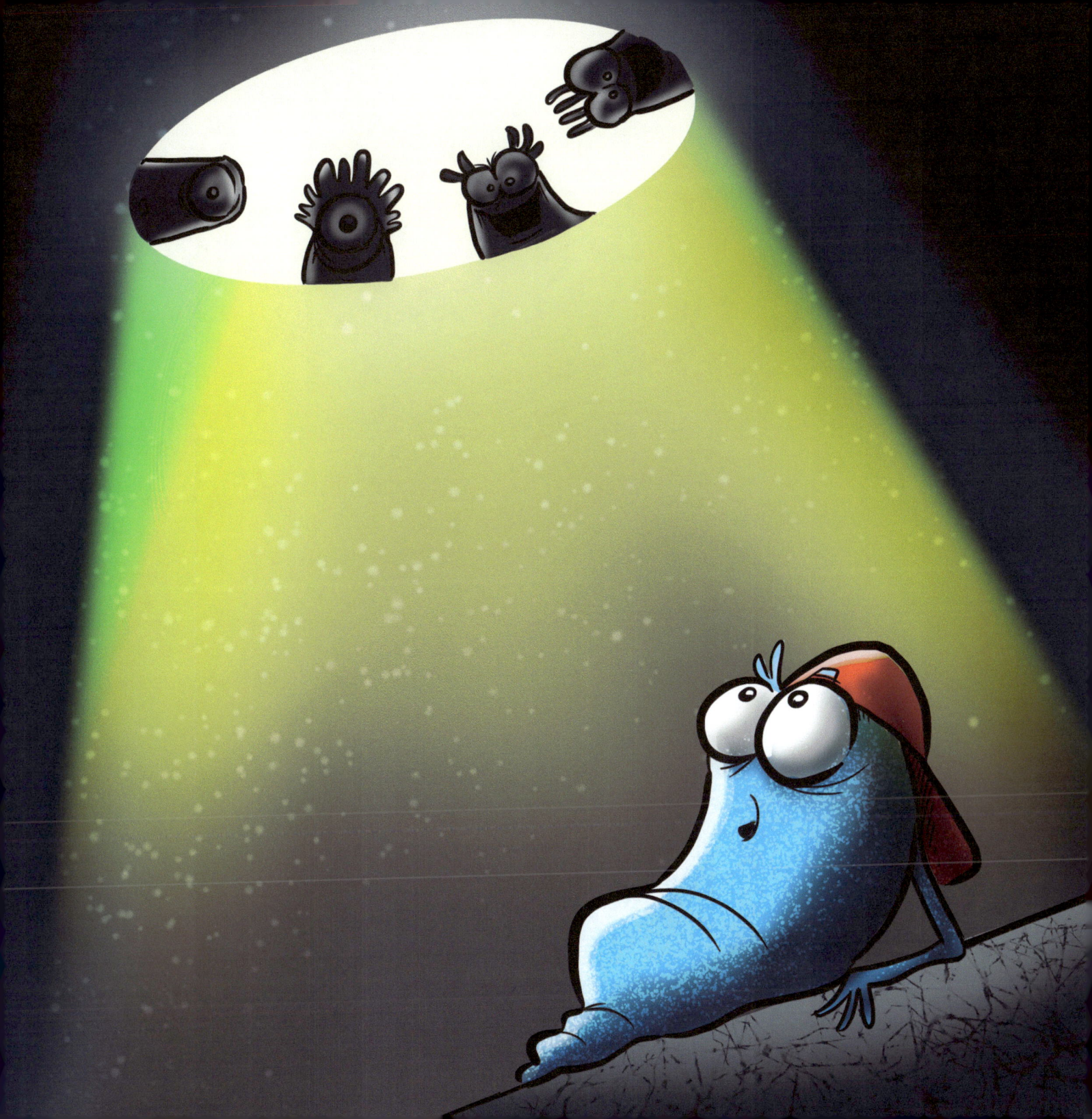

Mighty Bug felt safe and no longer alone.
He was happy the drain became his new home.
No people around to sneeze, sniffle, or cough.
No hand making stops to jump on or hop off.
All of the bugs remained safe in their chair.
No more sneezes to blast them through the air.

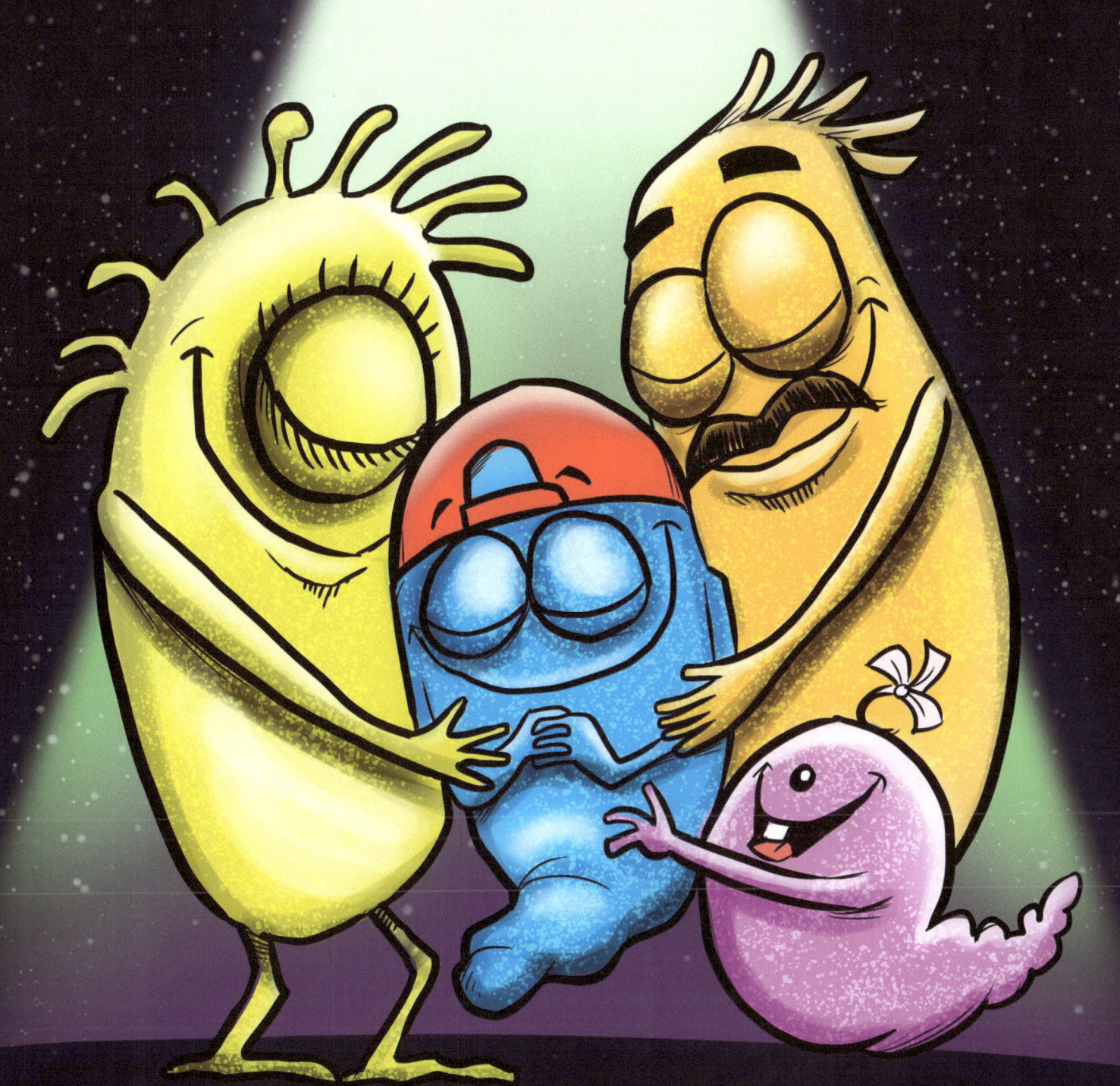

Mighty Bug called out from the drain to all the lands. He shouted to the people, "To keep us down here, just wash your hands!"

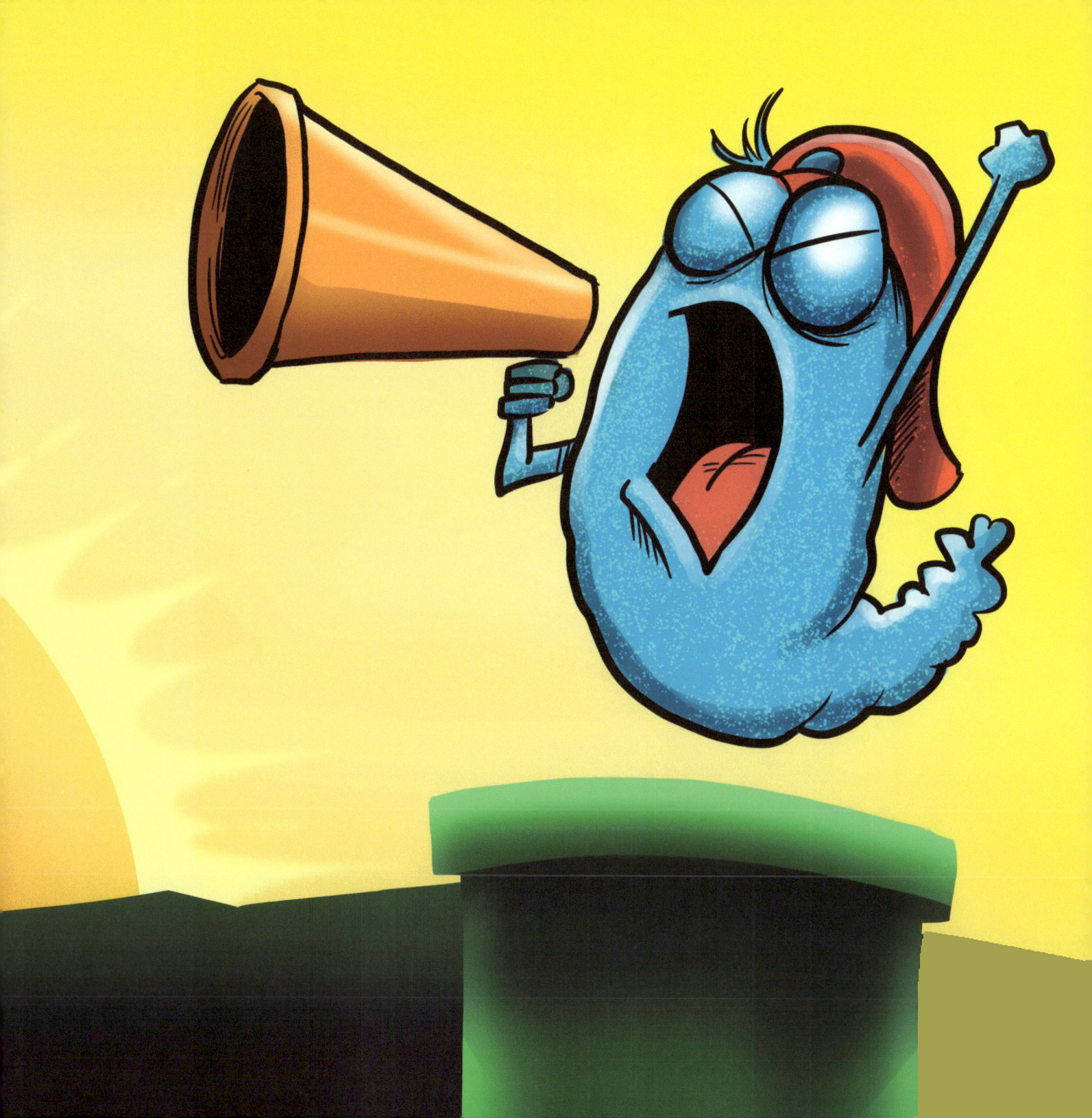

www.ingramcontent.com/pod-product-compliance
Lightning Source LLC
Chambersburg PA
CBHW041604120626
46551CB00002B/305